AIR FRYER COOKBOOK

2021

HEALTHY LUNCH AND SIDE DISH RECIPES
FOR BEGINNERS

JENNIFER WRIGHT

Table of Contents

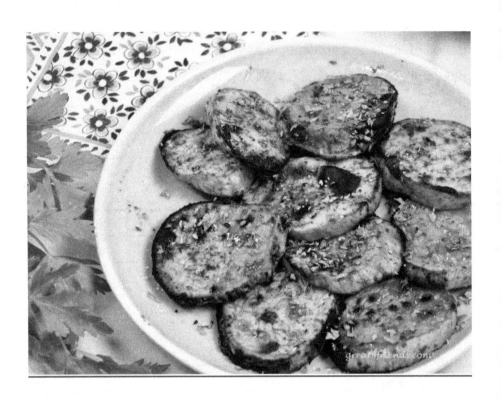

greatsblends.com

INTRODUCTION

All day we are running in a hurry to solve all the problems, earn more money and meet everyone we wanted – it seems like there is no place for the healthy ration. Sometimes we give up on this idea and start eating fast food. Sometimes we just can't find free minutes and hours to cook chicken meat in the oven or just roasted vegetables.

Moreover, we are wasting a lot of money on fast foods and lunches in restaurants. Air Fryer – it is effective solution of these problems. This is revolution in the food industry!

No more diets, no more wasting time and money. Forget about calories and weight – eat delicious food as usual, try new receipts every day and make your grey weekdays taste delicious.

Why cooking in Air Fryer is better? First of all, it doesn't take a lot of space. You can place this quite small (but still big enough to cook even whole chicken with honey) machine even in the small kitchen or office. Secondly, Air Fryer lets you cook without oil and this technology makes your ration several times healthier. Now you can finally forget about diets and stop starving to lose some weight.

Everything you cook in Air Fryer will be full of vitamins and low calories! It's hard to believe, but you can easily let yourself eat BBQ club sandwich with French fries and desserts and forget about additional pounds.

Air Fryer lets you economy both time and money. You don't need to add a lot of oil and look for complicated receipts. This small and easy to use machine will make all of your dreams come true.

This is your guide to the healthy life without diets and odd calories.

You will discover how it is easy and simple to cook delicious recipes to astonish your guest!

Lettuce Cups

No bread, no potato, only fresh lettuce with crispy bacon and melting cheese!

Prep time: 15 minutes

Cooking time: 15 minutes

Servings: 1

Ingredients:

- 1 strip bacon
- Parmesan
- Lettuce
- Cesar Dressing

Directions:

1. Turn on Air Fryer and preheat up to 340∘F.
2. Cut bacon into slices and place in the Air Fryer for 10 minutes.
3. Put fried bacon in the lettuce cups.
4. Cover lettuce with Parmesan.
5. Place cups into Air Fryer for 2 minutes.
6. Serve with Cesar Dressing!

Nutrition:

- Calories: 154
- Fat: 7g
- Carbohydrates: 16g
- Protein:7g

Mac & Cheese Wheel

This traditional Turkish pie can be perfect appetizer!

Prep time: 10 minutes

Cooking time: 30 minutes

Servings: 7

Ingredients:

- ½ cup sour cream
- Salt
- Pepper
- ½ cup milk
- ½ pound pasta
- ½ cup Gruyere cheese
- ¼ cup crumbs
- ½ cup Fontina cheese
- ½ cup cheddar cheese
- ¼ cup Parmesan cheese
- 1 tablespoon butter
- 1/8 cup nutmeg

Directions:

1. Turn on Air Fryer and preheat up to 350◦F.
2. Prepare separate boil with the hot water and boil pasta for 9 minutes.
3. When pasta is ready, cover it with the milk, all types of cheese from the list of ingredients, creams and salt with pepper and nutmeg. Mix well.
4. Form a circle and combine it with butter and nutmeg.
5. Put pasta circle into the Air Fryer and bake for 20 minutes.
7. Cut the pie and serve with basil.

Nutrition:

- Calories: 290
- Fat: 8g
- Carbohydrates: 38g
- Protein:17g

Masala Papad

This appetizer of papad is not only delicious, but nice-looking and easy to cook! It is easy to be healthy with Air Fryer!

Prep time: 10 minutes
Cooking time: 5 minutes
Servings: 1

Ingredients:

- 2 papads
- Green chili
- Onion
- ½ tomato

Directions:

1. Wash and cut tomato into the slices.
2. Make a mix of chopped onion and chili.
3. Halve each papad.
4. Turn on Air Fryer and preheat up to 360◦F.
5. Place papads in Air Fryer for 3 minutes.
6. Remove them from the Air Fryer and cover with vegetable mix.
8. Serve with olive oil.

Nutrition:

- Calories: 170
- Fat: 12g
- Carbohydrates: 12g
- Protein:3g

Meatloaf

This type of bread you will like for sure!

Prep time: 10 minutes

Cooking time: 25 minutes

Servings: 4

Ingredients:

- 4.4 pounds beef
- Breadcrumbs
- Onion
- Salt
- Pepper
- 3 tablespoons tomato ketchup
- 1 tablespoon herbs
- 1 teaspoon Worcester sauce
- 1 tablespoon parsley
- 1 tablespoon oregano
- 1 tablespoon basil

Directions:

1. Make a beef mince in the separate bowl.
2. Chop onion and mix it with the herbs, ketchup and sauce.
3. Add sauce with onion to the mince and mix well.
4. Turn on Air Fryer and preheat up to 340∘F.
5. Make a meatloaf of the mince with sauce and cover with crumbs.
6. Place meatloaf into the Air Fryer and cook for 25 minutes.
7. Serve with toasts and ketchup.

Nutrition:

- Calories: 279
- Fat: 17g
- Carbohydrates: 24g
- Protein:21g

Meatball Sandwiches

Roll up meatball sandwiches and get real pleasure!

Prep time: 10 minutes

Cooking time: 15 minutes

Servings: 2

Ingredients:

- 2 sandwich rolls
- Mozzarella cheese
- Cooked meatballs
- Pasta sauce

Directions:

1. Turn on Air Fryer and preheat up to 400°F.
2. Cover meatballs with pasta sauce and place into the Air Fryer for 5 minutes.
3. Add mozzarella cheese and cook for 5 more minutes.
4. Cut sandwich rolls.
5. Put sandwich rolls in the Air Fryer and cook for 2 minutes.
6. Place meatballs with cheese in the rolls.

7. Serve with ketchup sauce.

Nutrition:

- Calories: 416
- Fat: 12g
- Carbohydrates: 53g
- Protein:23g

Melting Mushrooms

Mushrooms filled with cheese and herbs – low calories and healthy lunch!

Prep time: 10 minutes

Cooking time: 10 minutes

Servings: 2

Ingredients:

- Olive oil
- Salt
- Pepper
- 10 button mushrooms
- Mozzarella cheese
- Cheddar cheese
- Herbs
- Drilled dill

Directions:

1. Wash and clean mushrooms.
2. Turn on Air Fryer and preheat up to 340∘F.
3. Make a marinade of olive oil, salt, pepper, herbs and dill. Cover mushrooms with the marinade.
4. Cut cheese on the small thin slices and mix Cheddar together with Mozzarella.
5. Fill mushrooms with cheese and place in the Air Fryer. Cook for 10 minutes.
6. Serve with the crumbs and Cesar sauce.

Nutrition:

- Calories: 275
- Fat: 16g
- Carbohydrates: 27g
- Protein:5g

Mini Cheese Scones

Out of time? Take quick and delicious lunch with you to the office!

Prep time: 5 minutes

Cooking time: 20 minutes

Servings: 10

Ingredients:

- 6.1oz flour
- Salt
- Pepper
- 0.88oz butter
- 1 teaspoon chives
- Egg
- 1 teaspoon mustard
- 1 tablespoon milk
- 2.6oz Cheddar cheese

Directions:

1. Turn on Air Fryer and preheat up to 340°F.
2. Make a mix of butter, flour and crumbs in the separate bowl.
3. Add Cheddar cheese and mix well.
4. Add milk and egg to get dough.
5. Put some flour on the table and form small balls of the dough.
6. Place leftover cheese on the dough balls and cook in the Air Fryer for 20 minutes.
7. Serve with sauce!

Nutrition:

- Calories: 396
- Fat: 19g
- Carbohydrates: 41g
- Protein:11g

Nacho Rolls

Really quick lunch to economy time and eat healthy food!

Prep time: 10 minutes

Cooking time: 15 minutes

Servings: 8

Ingredients:

- 1 pocket nacho balls
- Tomato sauce
- Egg
- 1 sheet puff pastry
- Sesame seeds

Directions:

1. Turn on Air Fryer and preheat up to 400 F.
2. Place nacho balls into the Air Fryer for 10 minutes.
3. Remove balls from the Air Fryer and cover each one with pastry.
4. Prepare plate with egg.
5. Place each ball into the egg and cover with sesame seeds.
6. Cook balls in Air Fryer for 10 minutes.

7. Serve with tomato sauce.

Nutrition:

- Calories: 150
- Fat: 8g
- Carbohydrates: 17g
- Protein:2g

Oregano Burgers

Two types of sauces, five types of herbs and fresh meat melting in your mouse together with vegetables – burgers can be not only delicious, but also healthy!

Prep time: 10 minutes
Cooking time: 10 minutes
Servings: 1

Ingredients:

- 1 tablespoon Worcestershire sauce
- Salt
- Pepper
- ½ teaspoon oregano
- 1-pound beef
- Liquid smoke
- 1 teaspoon parsley
- 1 teaspoon Maggi sauce
- ½ teaspoon onion powder
- ½ teaspoon garlic powder

Directions:

1. Turn on Air Fryer and preheat up to 350°F.
2. Make a mix of salt, pepper, garlic and onion powder with parsley and oregano.
3. Cover beef with seasoning and add liquid smoke.
4. Form burgers and put them into the hot Air Fryer.
5. Cook burgers for 10 minutes and add two types of sauces. Serve on the salad plate with salad of fresh vegetables.

Nutrition:

- Calories: 204
- Fat: 10g
- Carbohydrates: 5g
- Protein:22g

Pepperoni Quesadillas

Type of parshutto Italian pizza for you today!

Prep time: 15 minutes

Cooking time: 10 minutes

Servings: 4

Ingredients:

- 8 flour tortillas
- 1 can black olives
- 1 cup sliced mushrooms
- 8 slices mozzarella
- 1 jar pepperoni sauce
- ½ pepperoni
- Olive oil

Directions:

1. Turn on Air Fryer and preheat up to 375°F.
2. Prepare frying pan and warm up olive oil with mushrooms, olives and pepperoni.
3. Put on each tortilla half pepperoni sauce with filling and mozzarella.

4. Roll up pizza to close tortillas.

5. Place pizza rolls into the Air Fryer for 8 minutes.

6. Serve with fresh herbs.

Nutrition:

*   Calories: 465
*   Fat: 21g
*   Carbohydrates: 51g
*   Protein:20g

Pineapple Kebab

Do you want to add more vitamins to the ration? It's easy with this receipt!

Prep time: 10 minutes
Cooking time: 25 minutes
Servings: 1

Ingredients:

- 2 cups pineapple (in cubes)
- 2 ½ tablespoon sesame seeds
- 3 onions
- 3 eggs
- 5 chilies
- 3 tablespoons capsicum
- 1 ½ tablespoon ginger paste
- 3 tablespoons cream
- 1 ½ teaspoon garlic paste
- 4 tablespoons coriander
- Salt
- 2 teaspoons masala

- 3 teaspoons lemon juice

Directions:

1. Chop onion with coriander.
2. Turn on Air Fryer and preheat up to 340◦F.
3. Make a paste of masala, lemon juice, salt, pastes, seeds, capsicum and chilies.
4. Add onion with coriander to the mix.
5. Place pineapple cubes into the sauce.
6. Prepare separate plate with eggs.
7. Put each pineapple slice into the egg and place in the Air Fryer. Cook for 25 minutes.
8. Serve with crumbs and cheese.

Nutrition:

- Calories: 214
- Fat: 9g
- Carbohydrates: 19g
- Protein:13g

Poblano Chili Rings

Try to have truly healthy dinner quickly – this Mexican dish will be perfect lunch!

Prep time: 20 minutes

Cooking time: 25 minutes

Servings: 4

Ingredients:

- ½ cup crumbs
- ½ cup aquafaba
- ½ teaspoon salt
- 1 poblano chili

Directions:

1. Cut chili into the rings.
2. Turn on Air Fryer and preheat up to 390◦F.
3. Make a mix of crumbs with salt. Divide this mix on two parts.
4. Pour aquafaba on the clean plate
5. Place chili rings in aquafaba.
6. Put chili rings in crumbs mix.

7. Repeat procedure one more time.

8. Place rings into the Air Fryer and cook for 10 minutes.

9. Serve with toasts or soup.

Nutrition:

- Calories: 116
- Fat: 1,2g
- Carbohydrates: 22g
- Protein:4,5g

Pork Sandwiches

Fast food can be healthy – melting pork and fresh bread will make you satisfied and happy for the whole week!

Prep time: 20 minutes

Cooking time: 15 minutes

Servings: 4

Ingredients:

- 1 pork loin
- Salt
- Pepper
- ½ teaspoon garlic
- 4 buns
- ½ teaspoon red pepper
- Oil

Directions:

1. Turn on Air Fryer and preheat up to 350◦F.
2. Combine all spices in the separate plate.
3. Halve pork loin.
4. Cover pork with oil and seasoning.
5. Cook pork in the Air Fryer for 10 minutes.
6. Place buns in Air Fryer for 5 minutes more.
7. Put pork loin on the toasted buns and serve with berry sauce.

Nutrition:

- Calories: 361
- Fat: 15g
- Carbohydrates: 25g
- Protein:30,6g

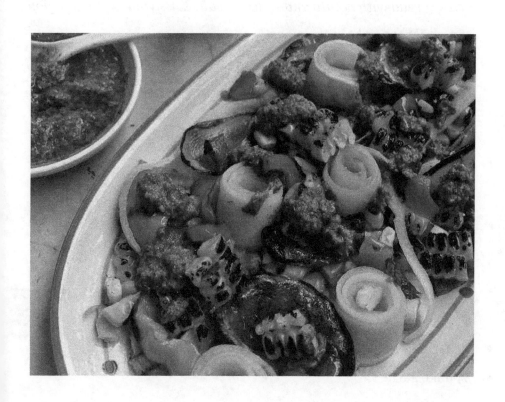

Potato Sandwich

Crispy bread with potato and sauce – really satisfying lunch, that you can easily eat right in the office!

Prep time: 10 minutes
Cooking time: 15 minutes
Servings: 2

Ingredients:

- 2 slices bread
- ¼ tablespoons chili sauce
- 1 tablespoon butter
- ¼ cup chopped onion
- ¼ flake garlic
- 1 capsicum
- Olive oil
- ¼ tablespoons Worcestershire sauce

Directions:

1. Turn on Air Fryer and preheat up to 300∘F.
2. Cut off edges of the bread slices.
3. Make a mix of garlic with olive oil, Worcestershire sauce, chili sauce and warm up on the frying pan.
4. Roast capsicum and cut into slices.
5. Add potato to the sauce and combine with capsicum.
6. Place mix into the bread and put sandwiches in the Air Fryer for 15 minutes.
7. Serve with cheese sauce.

Nutrition:

- Calories: 140
- Fat: 1,5g
- Carbohydrates: 26g
- Protein:6g

Pumpkin Parcels

Small and light mini pies will be perfect lunch for you both at home and in office!

Prep time: 5 minutes
Cooking time: 10 minutes
Servings: 9

Ingredients:

- Egg
- 3 tablespoons pumpkin filling
- 1 sheet pastry
- Flour

Directions:

1. Turn on Air Fryer and preheat up to 340∘F.
2. Put flour on the working surface. Cut pastry into the square slices.
3. Place pumpkin filling inside of each slice of pastry and roll up borders.
4. Cover borders with the beaten egg.
5. Place pastry into the Air Fryer and cook for 15 minutes.

6. Serve with fresh herbs.

Nutrition:

- Calories: 166
- Fat: 11g
- Carbohydrates: 14g
- Protein:4g

Ricotta Balls with Basil

Ricotta, seasoning and fresh herbs – all necessary for the healthy lunch full of vitamins!

Prep time: 10 minutes
Cooking time: 15 minutes
Servings: 1

Ingredients:

- 1 ½ cup of ricotta
- 3 slices white bread
- Pepper
- Salt
- ½ cup basil
- 2 tablespoons flour
- Egg
- 1 tablespoon chives

Directions:

1. Make a mix of egg yolk, flour, salt and pepper. Chop basil and chives. Add them to the mixture.
2. Cover ricotta with marinade.
3. Make balls of the mixture.
4. Turn on Air Fryer and preheat up to 400◦F.
5. Prepare one plate with egg white.
7. Take another plate and put crumbs on it.
8. Cover each ball with egg white and with crumbs.
9. Cook balls for 15 minutes.
10. Serve with cheese sauce.

Nutrition:

*   Calories: 215
*   Fat: 8g
*   Carbohydrates: 25g
*   Protein:9g

Roll up Lasagna

Everybody love lasagna! Eat it right on the work place – with this receipt it is possible!

Prep time: 15 minutes
Cooking time: 35 minutes
Servings: 12

Ingredients:

- 12 lasagna noodles
- 1 jar ragu sauce
- 15oz ricotta cheese
- 2 ½ cups mozzarella cheese
- Egg
- 2 teaspoons garlic
- 1 cup Parmesan
- Salt
- Pepper
- 1/3 teaspoon garlic salt
- 1/3 cup Romano cheese

Directions:

1. Turn on Air Fryer and preheat it up to 350∘F.
2. Take a special plate for your Air Fryer and cover with pasta sauce.
3. Cook lasagna noodles. Follow instruction on the pack.
4. Make a mix of ricotta with garlic. Add salt, pepper and egg. Mix well.
5. Add all the grated cheeses to the mix, apart mozzarella.
6. Lay lasagna sheets on the sauce on the plate for Air Fryer.
7. Place noodles above lasagna sheet and cover with sauce. Place meat sauce above.
8. Roll up every noodle and cover with mozzarella.
9. Place noodles into the Air Fryer and cook for 35 minutes.
10. Serve with fresh herbs.

Nutrition:

- Calories: 240
- Fat: 4g
- Carbohydrates: 22g
- Protein:13g

Salami Puffs

Perfect lunch is easy to take with you anywhere! Try this puffs: they are both satisfying and delicious

Prep time: 10 minutes
Cooking time: 15 minutes
Servings: 8

Ingredients:

- 1 salami
- Water
- Egg
- 3.5oz cream cheese
- 2sheets frozen pastry
- 2.8oz spinach

Directions:

1. Turn on air Fryer and preheat up to 400°F.
2. Clean salami of the skin and cut into cubes.
3. Make a mix of cheese with spinach in the separate bowl.
4. Cut pastry into the squares.

5. Place cream cheese in the center.

6. Put salami on top and roll pastry to get corners in the center.

7. Make a mix of egg with water and brush each pie with this mixture.

8. Place into the Air Fryer and cook for 10 minutes.

9. Serve with fresh herbs and ketchup.

Nutrition:

- Calories: 235
- Fat: 20g
- Carbohydrates: 2g
- Protein:10g

Sausage and Cheese Wraps

This is something healthier, more delicious and easier, than ordinary hot dogs – just try!

Prep time: 10 minutes

Cooking time: 10 minutes

Servings: 2

Ingredients:

- 8 sausages
- Ketchup
- 8 cheese slices
- 8 skewers
- 8 rolls dough

Directions:

1. Turn on Air Fryer and preheat up to 400∘F.
2. Place rolls on the dry working surface.
3. Cover each dough slice with cheese.
4. Put sausage on the dough.
5. Roll it up and put into the Air Fryer.

6. Cook rolls in Air Fryer for 5 minutes.
7. Cover with ketchup and serve.

Nutrition:

- Calories: 245
- Fat: 15g
- Carbohydrates: 13g
- Protein:21g

Shortbread Fingers

Only 15 minutes and delicious lunch on your table! This sweet and light bread fingers can be served both with cheese and with yogurt – make todays lunch special!

Prep time: 5 minutes

Cooking time: 15 minutes

Servings: 10

Ingredients:

- 6.1oz butter
- 8.8oz flour
- 2.6oz sugar

Directions:

1. Turn on Air Fryer and preheat it up to 340°F.
2. Make a mix of sugar and flour.
3. Place butter in the separate plate and warm up on the fire.
4. Add melting butter to the flour mixture.
5. Make fingers from the mixture and place into the Air Fryer.
6. Cook fingers for 15 minutes. Serve with creamy cheese or yogurt.

Nutrition:

- Calories: 170
- Fat: 9g
- Carbohydrates: 18g
- Protein:2g

Sliders

Let yourself a little bit more! For example, big and delicious slider! No extra calories and lots of vitamins – that's what you needed in your ration!

Prep time: 10 minutes

Cooking time: 10 minutes

Servings: 2

Ingredients:

- 8 slices beef
- 2 rolls
- Salt
- Pepper
- ¼ teaspoon garlic powder
- 2 cheddar cheese slices

Directions:

1. Turn on Air Fryer and preheat up to 390∘F.
2. Cut beef into slices and cover with salt, garlic and pepper.
3. Put beef in the Air Fryer and bake for 10 minutes.
4. Take beef, place on rolls and add some cheese inside of it.
5. Place burgers in Air Fryer and cook for 2 minutes.
6. Serve with ketchup.

Nutrition:

- Calories: 150
- Fat: 11g
- Carbohydrates: 3g
- Protein:12g

Stromboli

Now you can take this traditional Italian pizza with you wherever you want!

Prep time: 15 minutes

Cooking time: 20 minutes

Servings: 7

Ingredients:

- 1 can pizza dough
- 2 cups shredded mozzarella
- ½ cup pizza sauce
- 1 cup crumbled ground
- ½ cup sliced pepperoni
- Sausage
- Olive oil
- Parmesan
- Olives

Directions:

1. Turn on Air Fryer and preheat up to 400.F.
2. Prepare parchment paper.
3. Roll pizza dough on the parchment paper.
4. Boil sausage.
5. Put sauce with pepperoni and sausage on the dough. Cover with ground and mozzarella.
6. Roll up and place into the Air Fryer.
7. Make a mix of olive oil with parmesan and olives.
8. Place rolled pizza into the Air Fryer for 10 minutes.
9. Add cheese mix on top and cook 10 minutes more.
10. Serve with fresh herbs.

Nutrition:

- Calories: 385
- Fat: 29g
- Carbohydrates: 5g
- Protein:23g

Thai Fish Cakes with Mango Salsa

Dreaming about lunch full of vitamins? Let your dreams come true with this light and easy receipt!

Prep time: 10 minutes
Cooking time: 10 minutes
Servings: 1

Ingredients:

- 1 mango
- 1 ¾ coconut
- 1 ½ chili paste
- Onion
- Juice of 1 lime
- Egg
- 3 tablespoons coriander
- 1 white fish fillet

Directions:

1. Turn on Air Fryer and preheat it up to 380∘F.
2. Wash and cut mango into slices. Mix it with chili paste and lime juice.
3. Make a mix of egg, salt and mixture from the previous step and cover fish with it.
4. Cut onion into small cubes and mix fish in marinade with coconut, onion and coriander.
5. Form cakes from the fish mix.
6. Cook cakes in the Air Fryer for 7 minutes and cover with mango salsa.
7. Serve with coconut slices.

Nutrition:

- Calories: 282
- Fat: 10g
- Carbohydrates: 11g
- Protein:23g

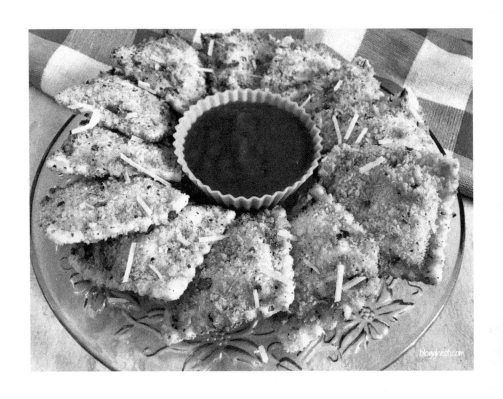

Toad in the Hole

One of the most popular dishes on the North of UK – try and you will love it!

Prep time: 10 minutes
Cooking time: 30 minutes
Servings: 4

Ingredients:

- 0.53oz rosemary
- 2 eggs
- 1 clove garlic
- 1 onion
- Cold water
- 5.8oz flour
- 8 sausages

Directions:

1. Take a small plate that will be suitable for your Air Fryer.
2. Put there olive oil, place flour above and add eggs to the mixture.
3. Add milk, water, garlic and onion to the mixture. Cover with salt and pepper.
4. Place sausages into the mixture and add rosemary leaves.
5. Turn on Air Fryer and preheat up to 340°F.
7. Bake sausages for half an hour.

Nutrition:

- Calories: 313
- Fat: 20g
- Carbohydrates: 22g
- Protein:15g

Welsh Rarebit

Traditional welsh toasts with cheese and eggs can both be perfect late breakfast and lunch full of vitamins!

Prep time: 10 minutes

Cooking time: 15 minutes

Servings: 2

Ingredients:

- 3 slices bread
- 4.2oz cheddar
- 2 eggs
- 1 teaspoon paprika
- 1 teaspoon mustard

Directions:

1. Turn on Air Fryer and preheat up to 340·F.
2. Place bread slices into the Air Fryer for 5 minutes.
3. Separate yolks from the egg whites.
4. Make a mix of egg yolks with cheese and paprika.
5. Add mustard and egg whites to the mix.

6. Pour this mixture on the bread slices into the Air Fryer and cook for 10 more minutes.
8. Serve with the berry sauce.

Nutrition:

- Calories: 164
- Fat: 13g
- Carbohydrates: 5g
- Protein:8g

SIDE DISHES

Avocado Fries

Ordinary French Fries seems to be ordinary dish already, but what about extra new receipt – avocado fries?

Prep time: 10 minutes
Cooking time: 10 minutes
Servings: 4

Ingredients:

- ½ cup crumbs
- Salt
- 1 avocado
- 1 Aquafaba

Directions:

1. Make a mix of crumbs with salt in the separate plate. It's better to use blender.
2. Turn on Air Fryer and preheat up to 390 F.
3. Mix blended crumbs with aquafaba.
4. Wash and peel avocado, cut into cubes.

5. Take one cube and place it in the crumbs mix. Repeat with all the other pieces.

6. Place cubes in Air Fryer for 10 minutes. Then shake them and bake for 5 minutes more.

7. Serve with creamy sauce and fresh herbs.

Nutrition:

- Calories: 51
- Fat: 5g
- Carbohydrates: 10g
- Protein:6g

Asparagus Salad

Warm salads – best way to have both healthy and delicious lunch!

Prep time: 10 minutes

Cooking time: 10 minutes

Servings: 4

Ingredients:

- 14.1oz asparagus (white – 8.8oz and green 5.1oz)
- 1 tablespoon olive oil
- 4 eggs (boiled)
- 2 mandarin oranges
- 2 red chicory
- 6 radishes
- 8.8oz potatoes
- 8.8oz salad leaves
- 8.8oz ham
- 8.8oz tomatoes

Directions:

1. Peel and boil potatoes in the bowl with hot salted water.
2. Turn on and preheat Air Fryer up to 400◦F.
3. Cut green and white asparagus.
4. Put olive oil, asparagus, ham and potatoes into the Air Fryer. Cook them for 10 minutes.
5. Leave prepared mixture to cool and add mandarin, radishes, salad and tomatoes.
7. Add salt and pepper to the salad. Mix well.
8. Add chicory and quarters of the boiled eggs. Serve this dish in salad deep plate with the olive oil.

Nutrition:

- Calories: 53
- Fat: 3g
- Carbohydrates: 7g
- Protein:2g

Baked Camembert with Soldiers

Crispy bread slices with melting and tender camembert – cheese pie for the lunch!

Prep time: 5 minutes
Cooking time: 15 minutes
Servings: 2

Ingredients:

- 1 camembert
- 2 slices bread
- Salt
- Pepper
- Fresh basil leaves
- Olive oil

Directions:

1. Turn on Air Fryer and preheat up to 340°F.
2. Cut bread into small stripes. Cover them with olive oil and cook in the Air Fryer for 5 minutes.
3. Place camembert on the frying pan for the Air Fryer.

4. Cook in Air Fryer for 15 minutes, then add bread slices and cook for 3 minutes more.
5. Cover with salt, pepper and serve with fresh basil leaves.

Nutrition:

- Calories: 285
- Fat: 22g
- Carbohydrates: 0,2g
- Protein:21g

Baked Mediterranean Vegetables with Crumbs

This is not a kind of ratatouille – this is boom of vitamins!

Prep time: 20 minutes

Cooking time: 45 minutes

Servings: 8

Ingredients:

- Olive oil
- 18oz of eggplant
- 4 garlic cloves
- 18oz of zucchini
- Thyme sprig
- 18oz of bell peppers
- Salt
- Pepper
- 4 onions
- Bay leaf
- 18oz of tomatoes
- Bread crumbs

Directions:

1. Turn on Air Fryer and preheat up to 380◦F.
2. Cut tomatoes and bake for 2 minutes.
3. Mix eggplant with olive oil and spices and cook for 4 minutes in Air Fryer.
4. Cook zucchini with olive oil in the Air Fryer for 4 minutes.
5. Finally, add tomatoes and bell peppers to the mix from the other vegetables and bake for 2 minutes more with olive oil and crumbs.
6. Serve in deep salad plate with cheese by the taste.

Nutrition:

- Calories: 279
- Fat: 13g
- Carbohydrates: 27g
- Protein:10g

Baked Shahi Tomatoes

East vibes for the lunch – try tender tomatoes with nuts and cheese!

Prep time: 10 minutes

Cooking time: 15 minutes

Servings: 3

Ingredients:

- 2 potatoes
- Salt
- 1.76oz cheese
- ½ teaspoon masala
- 2 tablespoons raisins
- 1 teaspoon coriander powder
- 3 tablespoons chopped cashews
- ½ teaspoon chili powder
- 2 tablespoons oil
- ¾ teaspoon ginger paste
- 1 teaspoon cumin seeds
- 2 chilies
- 2 tablespoon coriander leaves

- ¼ cup mozzarella

Directions:

1. Fry ghee on the frying pan for 3 minutes.
2. Chop chili peppers.
3. Add cumin seeds with ginger paste and chilies with powders on the frying pan.
4. Add cashews and raisins. Cook 3 more minutes.
5. Prepare bowl with hot water and boil potatoes.
6. Mash potatoes.
7. Mix potatoes with the mix on the frying pan.
8. Chop tomatoes.
9. Make tomatoes empty inside and fill with the mix from the frying pan.
10. Turn on Air Fryer and preheat up to 360°F.
11. Cover tomatoes with oil and cook for 10 minutes. Place cheese above and cook for 5 more minutes.
12. Serve with fresh basil leaves.

Nutrition:

- Calories: 206
- Fat: 12g
- Carbohydrates: 15g
- Protein:9g

Broccoli with yogurt

Broccoli can surprise you – just check out this new receipt!

Prep time: 35 minutes

Cooking time: 10 minutes

Servings: 2

Ingredients:

- 1 head broccoli
- 2 teaspoons lime juice
- 1 tablespoon oil
- 3 tablespoons powder
- 0.18oz mint
- 3 tablespoons salt
- 5.3oz Greek yogurt
- 0.18oz dill
- Salt
- Pepper
- Chopped mint leaves
- ½ onion
- 2 teaspoons sugar
- 3.4fl oz vinegar

- ½ teaspoons chili
- 0.18oz coriander
- 1 teaspoon blended garlic

Directions:

1. Mix sugar, salt, onion and chili. Place them on the simmer.
2. While spices are cooking, place on the simmer vinegar.
3. Add hot vinegar to the mixture.
4. Wait for 5 minutes until onion will be golden color.
5. Cut broccoli and add oil.
6. Turn on Air Fryer on 400ᵒF. Place broccoli into Air Fryer.
7. Bake broccoli for 12 minutes.
8. Mix yogurt with all the other ingredients.
10. Take out of the Air Fryer cooked broccoli and cover with the powder and salt.
11. Place yogurt on the plate – put in the center broccoli and cover with tomatoes.

Nutrition:

- Calories: 129
- Fat: 7g
- Carbohydrates: 12g
- Protein:6g

Brussels sprouts with Bacon and Cheese

Healthy food can be extremely delicious – try this side dish and make sure!

Prep time: 30 minutes

Cooking time: 5 minutes

Servings: 9

Ingredients:

- 3 pounds Brussels sprouts
- 1 cup milk
- 1 tablespoon thyme leaves
- 2 cups heavy cream
- 4 tablespoons flour
- Olive oil
- Salt
- Pepper
- 1 pound bacon
- 4 tablespoons butter
- ¼ tablespoon nutmeg
- 4 tablespoons horseradish
- 4 shallots
- Parmesan

Directions:

1. Turn on Air Fryer and preheat up to 400∘F.
2. Mix Brussels sprouts with olive oil and salt/pepper.
3. Bake Brussels sprouts in Air Fryer for 30 minutes.
4. Cook bacon – put it into the Air Fryer for 10 minutes. Add shallots and cook for 15 minutes more.
5. Make a mixture of melted butter, whisk and flour, add milk and creams to the sauce. Mix around 5 minutes.
6. Combine butter with horseradish, nutmeg and salt.
7. Change temperature in the Air Fryer to 350∘F.
8. Put Brussels sprouts in the Air Fryer, cover with sauce and place bacon above.
9. Bake Brussels sprouts for 30 minutes.
10. Serve the dish with the Parmesan on top and fresh herbs.

Nutrition:

- Calories: 130
- Fat: 5g
- Carbohydrates: 4g
- Protein:2g

Cauliflower Buffalo Bites

Fried vegetables can be delicious, but this easy receipt will make you fall in love with healthy food!

Prep time: 10 minutes

Cooking time: 20 minutes

Servings: 6

Ingredients:

- Salt
- Pepper
- Olive oil
- 1 tablespoon butter
- Hot sauce
- 1 head cauliflower
- 2 teaspoons garlic powder

Directions:

1. Cut cauliflower on slices.
2. Turn on Air Fryer and preheat up to 450°F.
3. Make a marinade of salt, pepper, olive oil and garlic powder.
4. Place pieces of cauliflower in the marinade for 15 minutes.
5. Cook cauliflower slices in the Air Fryer for 15 minutes.
6. Remove from the Air Fryer and cover with butter.

8. Bake cauliflower for 5 more minutes to get a golden skin.

Nutrition:

- Calories: 113
- Fat: 2g
- Carbohydrates: 20g
- Protein:6g

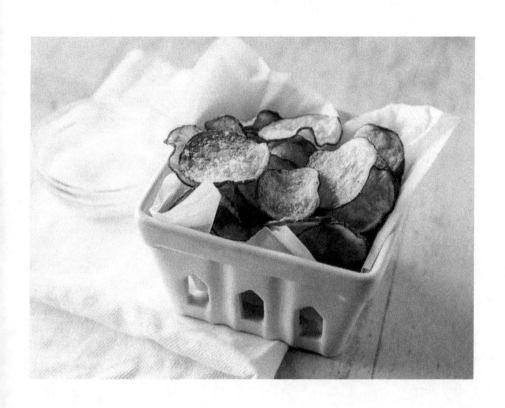

Cauliflower Stuffed Peppers

Even quick lunch in the office can be healthy! Stuffed peppers are easy to take with you and extremely delicious!

Prep time: 5 minutes

Cooking time: 20 minutes

Servings: 3

Ingredients:

- Green, yellow and red pepper
- Salt
- Pepper
- Cauliflower
- 1 teaspoon fennel seeds
- Onion
- 1 teaspoon coriander
- ¼ yellow pepper
- 1 teaspoon spice
- Carrot
- 1 teaspoon Chinese five spice
- Courgette

- Olive oil
- 1 teaspoon garlic puree
- 3 tablespoons soft cheese

Directions:

1. Turn on Air Fryer and preheat up to 400∘F.
2. Wash and clean peppers – remove all the seeds from inside.
3. Place empty peppers into the Air Fryer and cook for 5 minutes.
4. Prepare frying pan with olive oil and fry chopped onions with garlic. Cut vegetables and put on the frying pan. Fry for 5 minutes.
5. Add seasoning and cauliflower on the frying pan and cook for 3 more minutes.
6. Open Air Fryer and put some cream cheese inside, cover with cauliflower rice. Cook in Air Fryer for 10 more minutes.
7. Serve with the fresh basil leaves.

Nutrition:

- Calories: 78
- Fat: 2g
- Carbohydrates: 10g
- Protein:3g

Cheese Sticks

Light and delicious dish won't let you feel hunger for a long time!

Prep time: 5 minutes

Cooking time: 7 minutes

Servings: 5

Ingredients:

- Marinara sauce
- 12 pieces mozzarella cheese
- ¼ cup flour
- 2 cups bread crumbs
- 2 eggs
- ¼ cup Parmesan

Directions:

1. Put in the separate plates eggs, flour and mixture of Parmesan with breadcrumbs.
2. Turn on Air Fryer and preheat it up to 400∘F.
3. Take one piece of mozzarella and put it into the flour to be covered.
4. Put cheese into the egg.
5. Finish the procedure by placing mozzarella in the breadcrumbs.

6. Repeat procedure with all the mozzarella pieces.

8. Put mozzarella into the Air Fryer for 7 minutes.

9. In 7 minutes turn round every piece and leave it for 3 minutes more.

10. Serve this dish with the Cesar sauce.

Nutrition:

- Calories: 150
- Fat: 5g
- Carbohydrates: 17g
- Protein:10g

Cheesy Bacon Fries

Delicious and tender dish is perfect for your weekdays! Try bacon with cheese fries in Air Fryer – only few minutes and lunch is ready!

Prep time: 10 minutes

Cooking time: 10 minutes

Servings: 1

Ingredients:

- 1 potatoes
- Ranch dressing
- 5 bacon slices
- ¼ cup scallions
- Olive oil
- Salt
- Pepper
- 2 ½ cup Cheddar cheese
- 3 slices cream cheese

Directions:

1. Turn on Air Fryer and preheat up to 400∘F.
2. Boil potatoes.
3. Blanch potatoes and put into the cold water.
4. Cut bacon into slices and place it in the Air Fryer for 5 minutes.
5. Take bacon out of the Air Fryer and change temperature on 360∘F.
6. Place potato into the Air Fryer and cook for 25 minutes.
7. Mix Cheddar cheese with cream cheese.
8. Pour cheese mix on the potatoes and add bacon. Cover with salt and pepper.
9. Place mix into the Air Fryer and cook for 5 minutes.
11. Serve with fresh herbs.

Nutrition:

- Calories: 380
- Fat: 21g
- Carbohydrates: 39g
- Protein:8g

Coleslaw Pasta Salad

Try to add more Italian colors to the grey weekdays!

Prep time: 10 minutes

Cooking time: 15 minutes

Servings: 1

Ingredients:

- 4 slices bacon
- ½ cup cream
- 3 cups macaroni
- 1 cup mayonnaise
- ¼ cabbage
- Onion
- 2 carrots

Directions:

1. Prepare bowl with salted hot water and boil macaroni for 9 minutes.
2. Chop carrot and cabbage.
3. Turn on Air Fryer and preheat up to 400◦F.
4. Chop onion and place on the hot frying pan. Add carrot with cabbage and fry for 3 minutes.
5. Place macaroni with bacon to the Air Fryer for 5 minutes.
6. Add vegetables with cream and mayonnaise and cook for 7 minutes more.
7. Serve with fresh basil leaves.

Nutrition:

- Calories: 64
- Fat: 5g
- Carbohydrates: 3g
- Protein:1g

Courgette

Vegetables with cheese bakes in Air Fryer – healthy and extremely delicious dish!

Prep time: 10 minutes
Cooking time: 15 minutes
Servings: 4

Ingredients:

- Pepper
- 4 tablespoons cheese
- 2 courgettes
- 1 tablespoon oil
- 1 tablespoon chopped parsley
- 2 tablespoons breadcrumbs

Directions:

1. Turn on Air Fryer and preheat up to 340∘F.
2. Halve courgettes.
3. Blend cheese, oil, pepper, breadcrumbs and parsley.
4. Cover courgettes with the mix and cook in the Air Fryer for 15 minutes.

5. Serve dish on the flat plate with the sauce.

Nutrition:

- Calories: 16
- Fat: 1g
- Carbohydrates: 3g
- Protein:1g

Creamy Potato Soup

Light and satisfying soup it is the best variant to have quick and delicious lunch!

Prep time: 10 minutes

Cooking time: 30 minutes

Servings: 1

Ingredients:

- 4 potatoes
- 3.5oz cheese
- 2 cans chicken broth
- 1 pack cream cheese
- 1 can chicken soup
- Pepper
- ½ cup onion

Directions:

1. Wash and clean potatoes. Boil potatoes in the bowl.
2. Make a mix of the chicken with mashed potatoes and chopped onion. Add pepper. Blend it all together.
3. Turn on Air Fryer and preheat Air Fryer up to 340∘F.
4. Cook potatoes in the Air Fryer for 7 minutes.
5. Prepare bowl with the soup and cream cheese.
6. Add sauces and soup to the Air Fryer with potato and chicken and cook for 20 more minutes.
7. Add cheese on top of the soup.
8. Serve with fresh herbs.

Nutrition:

- Calories: 280
- Fat: 11g
- Carbohydrates: 40g
- Protein:5g

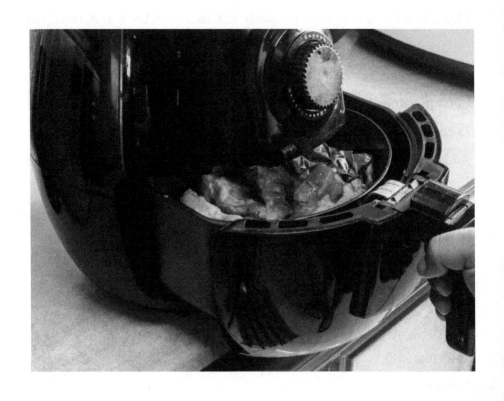

Crispy Tofu

Could you ever imagine – tofu can be as delicious as real meat? With Air Fryer it's true!

Prep time: 30 minutes

Cooking time: 20 minutes

Servings: 4

Ingredients:

- 1 block tofu
- 1 tablespoon potato starch
- Salt
- Pepper
- 2 teaspoons vinegar
- 2 teaspoons soy sauce
- 2 teaspoons olive oil
- Onion
- Basil

Directions:

1. Turn on Air Fryer and preheat up to 370∘F.
2. Open tofu and place on the separate plate.
3. Make a marinade of olive oil, vinegar and soy sauce.
4. Add spices to the marinade.
5. Cover tofu with marinade and wait for 10 minutes.
6. Cook tofu in the Air Fryer for 10 minutes.
7. Serve with fresh onion and basil.

Nutrition:

- Calories: 130
- Fat: 6g
- Carbohydrates: 15g
- Protein:9g

Crunchy Tofu

Tender tofu meat covered with crispy crumbles – in Air Fryer it is easy and quick to cook this dish!

Prep time: 15 minutes
Cooking time: 30 minutes
Servings: 4

Ingredients:

- 1 block tofu
- 1 teaspoon salt
- ¼ cup soy sauce
- ½ teaspoon garlic powder
- ½ cup mayo
- 1 cup crumbs
- 1 tablespoon oil
- 1 teaspoon ginger
- 1 teaspoon vinegar
- 1 tablespoon sesame oil

Directions:

1. Cut tofu into cubes.
2. Turn on Air Fryer and preheat up to 370∘F.
3. Make marinade of olive oil, sesame oil, soy sauce, garlic powder with ginger. Cover tofu with this marinade and leave for 20 minutes to rest.
4. Put mayo on the plate.
5. On another plate put mix of crumbs with salt.
6. Place each piece of tofu in mayo and in crumbs. Cook in Air Fryer for 20 minutes.
7. Serve with berry sauce.

Nutrition:

- Calories: 111
- Fat: 2g
- Carbohydrates: 26g
- Protein:4g

Faux Fried Rice

Green olives and tender meat – Greek vibes on the plate!

Prep time: 20 minutes

Cooking time: 40 minutes

Servings: 8

Ingredients:

- 1 tablespoon sesame oil
- ½ cup beaten eggs
- 1 tablespoon peanut oil
- 2 cans mushrooms
- 4 tablespoon soy sauce
- ¾ cup peas
- 4 cloves garlic
- Cauliflower
- 1 tablespoon ginger
- ½ lemon
- 1 can green olives

Directions:

1. Turn on Air Fryer and preheat up to 370◦F.
2. Make lemon juice and cut all the vegetables.
3. Make a mix of lemon juice, ginger, garlic, peas, soy sauce, oil and pour on the frying pan. Warm it up.
4. Blend cauliflower with chopped mushrooms and eggs.
5. Add sauce to cauliflower and mix well.
6. Place mix into the Air Fryer and cook for 25 minutes.
7. Serve with green olives.

Nutrition:

- Calories: 91
- Fat: 6g
- Carbohydrates: 6g
- Protein:4g

French Fries

Can fast food dish be healthy? Yes, now it can!

Prep time: 5 minutes

Cooking time: 30 minutes

Servings: 2

Ingredients:

- Oil
- 14oz peeled potatoes

Directions:

1. Cut potatoes to get stripes.
2. Fill the pan with the cold water.
3. Put potato slices into the water for 30 minutes. Add salt to the water.
4. Dry potatoes.
5. Spray slices with the oil.
6. Turn on Air Fryer and preheat it up to 350 F.
8. Place potato slices into the Air Fryer and wait for 30 minutes until it will be ready.

Nutrition:

- Calories: 197
- Fat: 11g
- Carbohydrates: 22g
- Protein:2g

Fried Tomatoes

Feel yourself lighter – try green tomatoes in bread crumbs!

Prep time: 5 minutes

Cooking time: 10 minutes

Servings: 1

Ingredients:

- 1 green tomato
- ¼ tablespoon of Creole seasoning
- Salt
- Pepper
- ¼ cup flour
- ½ cup buttermilk
- Bread crumbs

Directions:

1. Put flour on one plate. On the other plate place buttermilk.
2. Cut tomatoes and add salt with pepper.
3. Make a mix of seasoning with crumbs.
4. Take one tomato slices, cover with the flour, then place it into buttermilk, into crumbs and on the other plate. Repeat this procedure with all tomatoes.
5. Turn on Air Fryer and set temperature on 400∘F.
6. Cook tomato slices for 5 minutes.
7. Serve with basil.

Nutrition:

- Calories: 166
- Fat: 12g
- Carbohydrates: 11g
- Protein:3g

Garlic Tomatoes

Easy-cooking, nice-looking, light and healthy dish!

Prep time: 10 minutes

Cooking time: 15 minutes

Servings: 4

Ingredients:

- ½ teaspoon dried theme
- 4 tomatoes
- 1 clove garlic
- Salt
- Pepper
- 1 tablespoon olive oil
- 4 slices of bread

Directions:

1. Turn on Air Fryer and preheat up to 390°F.
2. Cover tomatoes with olive oil, salt, pepper, garlic and thyme.
3. Place tomatoes into the Air Fryer and fry for 15 minutes.
4. Put bread slices in the Air Fryer. Bake for 5 minutes.
5. Put tomatoes on the bread and cover with olive oil.

Nutrition:

- Calories: 152
- Fat: 6g
- Carbohydrates: 21g
- Protein:4g

Green Salad

Start your day with the healthy food! Green salad can empower you!

Prep time: 15 minutes

Cooking time: 10 minutes

Servings: 4

Ingredients:

- 1 lettuce
- 3 tablespoons yogurt
- 1 red bell pepper
- 1.8oz rocket leaves
- Black pepper
- 2 tablespoons olive oil
- 1 tablespoon lemon juice

Directions:

1. Turn on Air Fryer and preheat it up to 400∘F.
2. First of all, we need to prepare bell pepper. Just place it into the Air Fryer and wait for 10 minutes, until its skin become soft.
3. Cover bell pepper with the plastic wrap for 15 minutes and leave it.
4. Clean bell pepper and cut it.

5. Make a mixture from the lemon juice, olive oil, yogurt, salt and pepper. Add bell pepper.
6. Add lettuce and rocket leaves to the mixture and voila! Serve it in the big salad plate.

Nutrition:

- Calories: 15
- Fat: 0,2g
- Carbohydrates: 3,2g
- Protein:0,9g

Grilled Ham in Cheese

Grilled tender meat in light creamy cheese – that's the dish, that will make you satisfied for all the day!

Prep time: 10 minutes
Cooking time: 5 minutes
Servings: 2

Ingredients:

- 4 slices bread
- ¼ cup butter
- 2 slices ham
- 2 slices cheese

Directions:

1. Turn on Air Fryer and preheat up to 360◦F.
2. Cover one side of the bread slice of butter.
3. Repeat procedure with all slices.
4. Lay cheese on the bread and cover with ham. Close sandwich with another bread slice.
5. Place sandwich in Air Fryer and cook for 5 minutes.

6. Serve with Cesar sauce.

Nutrition:

- Calories: 230
- Fat: 13g
- Carbohydrates: 21g
- Protein:3g

Grilled Vegetables with Lamb

Both healthy and delicious dinner – grilled vegetables with roasted lamb! Spices and olive oil will add something special to this dish!

Prep time: 3 hours
Cooking time: 20 minutes
Servings: 2

Ingredients:

- 4 lamb slices
- Mint
- Rosemary
- Pepper
- Salt
- 1 carrot
- Olive oil
- 1 purple carrot
- 1 parsnip
- 1 fennel bulb

Directions:

1. Cut vegetables and put them into the water.
2. Mix mint and rosemary. Chop them together.
3. Place vegetables into the olive oil (we will need around 3 tablespoons) and add some salt with pepper.
4. Cover lamb slices with marinade and leave them for 3 hours to rest.
5. Turn on Air Fryer and preheat it up to 400◦F.
7. First of all, put lamb into the Air Fryer for 2 minutes.
8. In 2 minutes add vegetables and bake for 6 minutes more.
9. Serve with brunches of rosemary.

Nutrition:

- Calories: 385
- Fat: 7,7g
- Carbohydrates: 28g
- Protein:20g

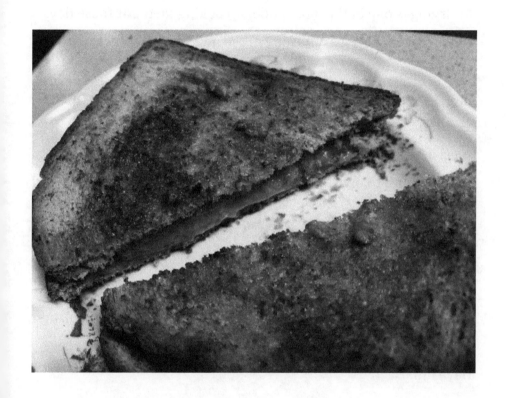

Conclusion

Air frying is one of the most popular cooking methods these days and air fryers have become one of the most amazing tools in the kitchen.

Air fryers help you cook healthy and delicious meals in no time! You don't need to be an expert in the kitchen in order to cook special dishes for you and your loved ones!

You just have to own an air fryer and this great air fryer cookbook!

You will soon make the best dishes ever and you will impress everyone around you with your home cooked meals!

Just trust us! Get your hands on an air fryer and on this useful air fryer recipes collection and start your new cooking experience!

Have fun!